Healthy Living

Lose Weight with Rejuvenating Smoothies

25 Best Smoothie Recipes Ever!

Madison Miller

DISCLAIMER

TABLE OF CONTENTS

SUMMARY

Thank you for buying **Lose Weight with Rejuvenating Smoothies, and 25 Best Smoothie Recipes Ever!** In here, you'll find secrets to losing weight naturally and becoming more youthful and fit as you age. It's all about smoothies! Smoothies are great to help you lose weight. They are THE way to create low-calorie, nutrient-rich meals. You get all the ingredients you want because YOU decide which ones you want. Meals-in-a-glass! They keep you full for a long time, so there's less chance of you needing to snack. And hey, if you want to snack, you can have another smoothie because they're so low in calories! Included in this book are great combinations of flavors, protein, healthy carbs and fats, and vitamins and minerals to make the smoothies you want! There are 25 great smoothie recipes in this book to aid you in your quest for weight-loss!

If you're ready to learn the magic of gaining health and losing weight as soon as possible, let's get on with it! Here we go!

INTRODUCTION

Smoothies for Weight Loss and Great Health

Let's face it, no drink or food guarantees instant weight loss – not even a rich, nutrient-dense smoothie. In order to lose weight and experience great health transformation, one of things you need to do is to eat fewer calories with better food. Since most smoothies are made from several "super foods" and are low in calories, drinking smoothies as a substitute for unhealthy food options is one of the best strategies you can choose for successful weight loss. This is the fact that makes smoothies a natural and smart way to lose weight. You also have to burn more calories than you consume, but if you're drinking smoothies like these instead of eating chips and cream puffs, you'll have to do much less at the gym!

Smoothies and Your Weight Loss Goal

The term "smoothie" can be used for a variety of beverages. Of course, some use better ingredients and are thus healthier than others. Really healthy smoothies contain one or more super foods that not only help you lose weight, but also provide you with nourishment that keeps you healthy, active, and rejuvenated.

Most of these smoothies contain fresh leafy greens, which makes them super healthy and gives them their "interesting" hue. The ingredients in these smoothies come from a large variety of foods, flavors, and colors. Most of them contain a mixture of green vegetables, healthy fruits, and possibly oils, dairy, and other ingredients. All the veggies and fruits are high in fiber, and we all know that the consumption of dietary fiber is inversely linked with body weight and body fat content. Thus, adding them to your diet in the form of smoothies is an easy, key method to aid weight loss.

According to surveys, drinking smoothies not only adds a variety of flavors in your diet, but also is one of the best ways to lose weight without starving yourself or having to prepare low-calorie meals three times a day. In short, smoothies provide nutrition, minerals, vitamins, fiber, healthy carbohydrates, and low-fat whole foods/super foods that you require in order to lose weight safely, quickly and effectively, without following strict diets that force you to starve yourself.

So How Do Smoothies Help Lose Weight?

If prepared following the right directions, smoothies can satisfy your hunger and help keep you from feeling hungry for a quite a while. Since they are loaded with healthy foods, you can easily replace your meals with a glass of a healthy smoothie.

In dieting, skipping meals to reduce weight is considered unhealthy and short-sighted. In this diet, you will replace your meals with low-calorie, high-nutrition, super food liquid, which can work wonders for you. It will become your most effective strategy to minimize the consumption of calories while still getting all the important sustenance for your body, AND all coming from vegetables and fruits.

A diet that includes smoothies is a preferable choice for many folks because it is easy to follow, far less complicated than other diets, and the end results are worth appreciating. As always, before starting any diet, check with your doctor to see if it's a good one for you.

The smoothie recipes shared in this book are not like the expensive smoothies available in the market. In fact, those smoothies are often loaded with all kinds of sweeteners and sugar that can defeat your main goal of losing weight. The solution for getting better smoothies is to make yourself at home. There are 25 weight-loss smoothies recipes shared in this book for you to try. Once you get the basic idea of making a healthy smoothie, you can always come up with your personalized variations of smoothies that not only serve your taste buds, but also help you with your weight loss goals.

SMOOTHIES – IS THAT MY WEIGHT LOSS SOLUTION?

The answer to that question is very probably yes, with a couple of conditions.

First, you must know what you have in your smoothie. Is it a perfect blend of super foods, healthy veggies, fruits, and whole foods, or is it loaded with sugar and unhealthy sweeteners for flavor? There is a reason why nutritionists and health experts suggest people prepare their own smoothies with 100% natural or organic ingredients instead of buying smoothies from supermarkets. The fact that many of the smoothies in your local grocery have either sugar on artificial sweeteners in them bears repeating! They're no good!

Homemade smoothies are full of ingredients that YOU choose. The ones in this book have natural sources of protein, healthy and filling carbohydrates, and healthy fats, made from nutritious fruits, energizing greens, and other delicious and natural ingredients.

My Daily Smoothie Consumption

So how many smoothies should I consume in a day? While following the smoothie diet, the key is to make sure you don't allow yourself to become hungry often. If you do get hungry, don't fulfill your cravings with unhealthy food. Instead drink another smoothie, and stop when you start feeling full! Don't worry if you're drinking smoothies more than three times in a day. You'll still lose weight.

Explaining Detox Symptoms

Some people may experience a few detox symptoms such as tiredness, headaches, and weakness. This is for a couple reasons. One, because you'll be taking a break from consuming your regular (maybe unhealthy) food, your body will try be yelling for you to feed it what it wants. Sugar and simple carbs are not happy when they stop getting fed. Don't worry, you'll get through it. It only lasts for a few days, and if you keep your eye on the prize of losing weight and switching to great foods, it will be a snap! To effectively achieve your weight loss goal and improve your smoothie diet, cut yourself off sweeteners such as brown sugar, white sugar, maple syrup, and honey from the ingredients. In addition to giving the sweet flavor, these ingredients provide you with unneeded calories and have very poor nutritional value. To add natural sweetness to your smoothies, try adding sweet fruits. They are a good, healthy source of sugar that can be used in smoothies.

Second, if you try to drink all smoothies for a few days, you'll be drinking liquids almost entirely, so frankly, you'll be expelling mostly liquids. While this is nothing to fear, if you do feel sick following this diet, you should stop and consult your health specialist. Better yet, follow our advice above, and talk to your doctor before you start it. Of course, you can also just try incorporating one or two smoothies into your regular diet.

Smoothie Recipe Tips

It is, of course, best to prepare your smoothies from natural and organically grown vegetables and fruits. You will certainly want to expand your smoothie possibilities and explore a wide variety of veggies and fruits to use. Include as many great foods as you can in a blend for maximum weight loss and health benefits.

Whenever possible, try to add the following in your diet: spinach, avocados, cucumber, mangos, pineapple, bananas, peaches, nectarines, and apples. These are some of the best assortments for preparing smoothies for weight loss.

Tip 1 – Add More Proteins to Your Smoothies

Load your smoothie cup with protein by adding more natural yogurt, dairy products, protein powder, or whey protein. These proteins are not only great for achieving your weight loss goal, but are crucial for repairing muscles. Moreover, adding protein to your smoothies helps to fill you up more so that you feel satisfied and don't feel the need of consuming more food.

Tip 2 – Add Fiber to Your Smoothies

Food items loaded with fiber like vegetables, nuts, oatmeal, whole wheat, and fruits can boost digestive tract health, cure bloated stomach, and stop irregular bowel problems. Vegetables, green beans, and fresh apples are a fantastic way to add dietary fiber to your daily consumption.

Tip 3 – Your Smoothies Should be Calcium-Rich

According to research, foods that are rich in calcium – including milk products or low-fat dairy products – are effective in reducing the chances for a person to develop heart problems and obesity.

With all of that information now tucked nicely in your head, let's get on to the fun part – the recipes! Get the blender out, tie your apron on, and let's get busy!

THE RECIPES

Citrusy-Creamy Fat-Burning Smoothie

This smoothie recipe for weight loss is the perfect blend that can be used as a meal replacement to help you achieve your goal of a slimmer body. The ingredients for this recipe will fill you up, control your cravings, boost your metabolism, and help you burn fat – all at the same time! The main ingredients, including coconut, avocado, grapefruit, and lemons, are loaded with nourishment that not only helps in weight loss but also keeps you healthy and revitalized.

Nutritional Values per Serving
Calories: 483
Total Fat: 28g
Carbohydrates: 56g
Protein: 12g

Ingredients
2 cups green tea (cooled)
½ can coconut milk,
¼ cup pitted dates (about 4 dates)
½ avocado (cored and peeled)
½ grapefruit (red preferred)

juice of 1 lemon

1 cup spinach (tightly packed)

3 bananas (medium-sized)

2 - 4 drops grapefruit therapeutic grade essential oils,

Preparation Method

Blend the liquid and the dry ingredients in a high speed blender for a minute (keep greens aside). Next, add the greens to the blender, and pulse again to combine all ingredients.

Add the fruits and the remaining ingredients, and blend until smooth. Add the essential oils in the end. Give it one last spin before serving it in a glass.

Tips: This is the ideal blending method, as it allows the dry ingredients to blend multiple times. Make sure you blend the dry with the liquids first, and then add the remaining ingredients. Also, you can use a little water if the smoothie appears to be too thick. You can use any other ingredients instead of bananas at the end to use it as fillers. Add ice, and chill the smoothie before serving.

Passion Fruit and Mango Smoothie

This amazing tropical blend of fruits is the perfect beverage to start your day the nutritious way – loaded with essential vitamins and low in fat. The best thing about this fruity smoothie is that it is absolutely sweetener free and nut free. It is literally only fruits. You have the flexibility of turning this fruit smoothie into a green one by using optional ingredients including oats and spinach. So check out the recipe and give yourself a much-needed nutrient boost!

Nutritional Values per Serving

Calories: 121

Total Fat: 1g

Carbohydrates: 23g

Protein: 6g

Ingredients

1 cup apple juice

1 cup orange juice

1 medium-sized mango (peeled and chopped)

1 banana

1 passion fruit

juice of 1 lime

1 cup spinach, (optional)

1 cup oats, (optional)

Preparation Method

Add all the ingredients in the juicer along with the liquid. and pulse for a short time (leaving out the oats and greens). Add the greens next along with the oats (if using), and blend again to combine. Blend until all ingredients are combined well and smooth.

Pour in your favorite smoothie mug and enjoy. If you like a chilled smoothie, don't hesitate adding a few ice cubes before you drink it down!

Tips: Add water to your smoothie to adjust the consistency if you like. You can add more and varied fruits to give this recipe a personalized touch.

Rippled Red-Berry Smoothie

The Rippled Red-Berry Smoothie is a very flavorful and exotically colored smoothie that you can enjoy at any time of the day. Not only is the recipe nutritionally rich, the flavors of fresh or frozen raspberries give this smoothie a fantastic taste. The natural flavor of this amazing, weight-loss smoothie is creamy and sweet and will fill you up instantly.

Nutritional Values per Serving
Calories: 279
Total Fat: 13g
Carbohydrates: 43g
Protein: 4g

Ingredients
1½ cups water
½ cup coconut milk
¼ cup pitted dates (about 4 dates)
2 cups raspberries
1 cup mango
1 cup oats, (optional)

Preparation Method
Add all the fruits along with the water and coconut milk in the blender or juicer and pulse on high for a short time to

combine all the ingredients together. Add oats (if using and pulse again. Keep blending until it forms a thick, creamy smoothie.

Don't forget to add the final raspberry ripple swirl to your smoothie. Pour your smoothie in a glass, and swirl a teaspoon of additional coconut milk in the middle of the smoothie. Chill your smoothie with ice cubes and enjoy.

Dreamy-Creamy Green Orange Smoothie

This blend of whole foods does not require milk or any other dairy alternative to make. The smoothie is not only rich in essential nutrients, it is creamy, flavorful, and bright green with a hint of fresh orange flavor. Prepare and try it yourself.

Nutritional Values per Serving

Calories: 156

Total fat: 2g

Carbohydrates: 32g

Protein: 3g

Ingredients

1 orange (peeled)

1 medium-sized zucchini

½ cucumber (peeled)

½ cup oats, (optional)

¼ cup cashews

1 scoop protein powder, (optional)

Note: In case you are not using vanilla protein powder, use ¼ teaspoon of vanilla.

Preparation Method

Add the fruits and vegetables in a blender, and blend to combine the juices. Add cashews, oats (if using), and protein powder (or vanilla), and blend again until the texture of your fruity smoothie is rich and creamy.

Pour into your favorite glass and enjoy the refreshing flavors of fresh fruits and veggies.

Banana Pie and Sweet Potato Smoothie

Banana Pie and Sweet Potato Smoothie is a perfect blend of whole foods and flavorful ingredients that are sugar free, gluten free, free from oats, and vegan. For those of you who want to gain maximum nutrients from a smoothie and are intolerant to oats, you can definitely try this one for weight loss and other health benefits. Prepare this one with confidence because it tastes exactly like sweet pie!

Nutritional Values per Serving
Calories: 358
Total Fat: 11g
Carbohydrates: 68g
Protein: 5g

Ingredients
1½ cups water
1 cup sweet potato (cooked or raw)
4 cups bananas
½ cup raisins
¼ cup pecans
1 teaspoon cinnamon
¼ cup coconut (dried)
1 cup spinach

Preparation Method

Add spinach and water in the blender, and blend to juice. Add all the remaining ingredients to your blender, and pulse again to combine all with the green juice and make a thick smoothie.

You can add more water to adjust the consistency of your smoothie. Add some ice cubes to your blender, and blend for a few seconds to crush the ice and enjoy chilled.

Zucchini Bread Smoothie

Zucchini is an amazing veggie that blends perfectly with smoothies, puddings, and sweet breads. Low in calories, zucchini can make your smoothie creamy and give it a very unique, interesting flavor. Since zucchini is low in calories, it makes the perfect ingredient for your weight loss smoothie. Serve yourself a glass of zucchini bread smoothie and feel energized and refreshed.

Nutritional Values per Serving

Calories: 289

Total Fat: 11.1g

Carbohydrates: 37.7g

Protein: 11.9g

Ingredients

2 cups milk (dairy free)

2 cups zucchini (chopped)

2 cups bananas

¼ cup pecans

¼ cup pitted dates (about 4 dates)

1 teaspoon ground vanilla/vanilla extract

1 teaspoon cinnamon

A pinch of sea salt

1 cup spinach, (optional)

Preparation Method

In case you are using spinach in this smoothie, blend it first with dairy-free milk in a blender. Add all the remaining ingredients, and pulse to combine, making a smooth mixture. Add more milk to adjust the consistency if you like.

Add ice and blend for a few seconds to enjoy smoothie with crushed ice. Drink immediately, and enjoy the fresh flavors.

Pear and Almond Smoothie

The recipe uses whole almonds and pears to make the perfect, delicious blend. While the texture of this smoothie isn't as smooth as you may like, the unique taste will balance out everything! Prepare this nutritionally rich smoothie that will greatly help you with your weight loss goal. No one can stop you from enjoying this smoothie!

Nutritional Values per Serving

Calories: 369

Total Fat: 12g

Carbohydrates: 67g

Protein: 6g

Ingredients

2 cups almond milk

4 cups pears

¼ cup almonds

1 cup spinach, (optional)

Preparation Method

If you are using the spinach, blend it with the almond milk first before adding any other ingredient. This will help you have more space in your blender before continuing on. Add the remaining two ingredients in the blender next, and pulse until it forms a thick, gritty mixture.

Add more milk to adjust the consistency if you like. Pour in a glass, add some ice cubes and serve immediately.

Frozen Orange and Pineapple Smoothie

The hint of pineapple and orange will not only give this amazing smoothie the best of flavors, but are also the nutrient-rich fruits great for your weight loss and your overall well-being. The blend of raw fruits and vegetables is what makes this smoothie refreshing and mouth-watering. Try it out yourself!

Nutritional Values per Serving

Calories: 265

Total Fat: 1g

Carbohydrates: 67g

Protein: 3g

Ingredients

1½ cups orange juice

3 cups pineapple

1 banana

1 tablespoon lime juice

1 cup oats, (optional: if you want to make a thick fruit smoothie)

1 cup spinach, (optional: to make it a green smoothie)

Preparation Method

Blend the spinach (if you are using it) first with orange juice or some water. Now add all the remaining ingredients (except the optional oats) in the green juice, and blend to combine well. Pulse until it forms a thick, creamy mixture. Add oats, and give it a final, long blend to combine well and form a thick smoothie.

Pour in a glass, and add crushed ice from the top. Serve immediately to taste the fresh flavors of all the ingredients. The hint of orange and pineapple flavors makes this smoothie a very delicious option for your weight loss. Must try!

Spiced Butternut Raw Squash Smoothie

Butternut Squash Smoothie is prepared with two types of non-dairy milk, raisins, and bananas for sweetening and texture, and nutmeg and cinnamon for the spicy touch. All the ingredients in this smoothie will make a great blend that serves you with a high level of nutrition and great taste!

Nutritional Values per Serving
Calories: 324
Total Fat: 7.5g
Carbohydrates: 67g
Protein: 4g

Ingredients
½ cup coconut milk
1½ cups milk (non-dairy) (oat, soya, rice, hemp, almond, raw nut, coconut drink or seed milk)
1 cup spinach
½ cup
2 cups raisins, butternut squash
1 teaspoon vanilla
6 bananas
½ teaspoon cinnamon
¼ teaspoon ground nutmeg

Preparation Method

Add the liquids to the blender along with the spinach.

Pulse the blender at high to prepare the green juice first.

Add all the remaining ingredients next, and blend again to form a rich and creamy smoothie.

You can add more milk to adjust the consistency of your smoothie. Add ice, and give it one final blend for a few seconds to crush the ice. Serve chilled immediately for maximum nutrients and best flavors.

Enjoy every sip of it!

Turbo Nutrient-Booster Smoothie

Just as the name suggests, the list of high-vitamin vegetables used in this smoothie will definitely give you the much-needed nutrient boost. Not only is the smoothie amazing for weight loss, the vegetables provide ample amounts of vitamins and minerals for the body.

Nutritional Values per Serving

Calories: 324

Total Fat: 12g

Carbohydrates: 42g

Protein: 5g

Ingredients

½ cucumber

1 tomato

½ clove garlic

1/8 onion

1 stalk celery

½ avocado

¼ romaine lettuce head

¼ teaspoon turmeric

20 mint leaves

juice of ½ lemon

a handful of parsley

1 teaspoon ginger (fresh or dried)

1 pinch cayenne pepper/chili powder

1 cup ice

Preparation Method

Chop the tomato, cucumber, onion, garlic, celery, lettuce, avocado, parsley, and ginger. Add all the ingredients to the blender, and pulse to combine well, until it forms a creamy smoothie. While the tomato and cucumber will provide all the liquid to form the smoothie, you may add more if you like to adjust the consistency. Blend at high speed for 3-4 minutes to ensure the bits and pieces of the vegetables are not left out.

Add ice and blend again until it crushes down and mixes with the remaining ingredients. Serve immediately, and enjoy chilled for great flavors.

Berries and Raw Buckwheat Smoothie

The raw buckwheat together with bananas and berries is filling and creamy. It's low in calories and rich in antioxidants and omegas. If you want a nutrient-booster smoothie, look nowhere else, because this is exactly what you are looking for!

Nutritional Values per Serving

Calories: 213

Total Fat: 8g

Carbohydrates: 15g

Protein: 6g

Ingredients

1/3 cup raw buckwheat (soaked in water for at least 30 minutes)

¼ cup almond milk

½ cup raspberries (frozen or fresh)

¼ cup strawberries (frozen or fresh)

1 tablespoon lemon juice

1 small-sized cucumber (peeled)

¼ cup pitted dates (about 4 dates)

1 teaspoon vanilla

½ avocado

small piece of ginger

Preparation Method

Place all the ingredients in a high-speed blender one by one, and pulse to combine until nice and smooth. Taste and adjust the ingredients to personalize flavors. The berries will give this delicious smoothie its rich color, while the ingredients will make it effective for your weight loss and overall well-being.

Sweet Romaine Lettuce Smoothie

With the wide range of delicious and wholesome ingredients, sweet romaine lettuce smoothie is a must-have for your smoothie diet plan. The beverage is low in calories and loaded with nutrients that boost your metabolism and aid weight loss successfully.

Nutritional Values per Serving

Calories: 287

Total Fat: 7g

Carbohydrates: 5g

Protein: 3g

Ingredients

1 cup water

1 cup milk (dairy free)

1 cup strawberries

1 banana or mango

1 apple (chopped)

1 cup pineapple

1 cup romaine lettuce (chopped)

2 tablespoons pumpkin seeds

½ cup apricots (dried)

1 cup oats

Preparation Method

Add the romaine lettuce and water to the blender, and pulse to combine. Add all the remaining ingredients to the blender (except oats) and blend at high until it forms a creamy mixture.

Add oats next, and give it another high-speed pulse to combine well. Adjust the consistency of your smoothie by adding more dairy-free milk if you like. Add ice cubes and give your smoothie a final pulse.

Serve immediately and enjoy!

Nutritional Key Lime-Pie Smoothie

The mixture of lime, dates, and fruits makes this smoothie a super hit. Combine these nutrient-rich ingredients together to form a smoothie that aids in weight loss and helps you maintain optimum health.

Nutritional Values per Serving

Calories: 318

Total Fat: 13g

Carbohydrates: 13g

Protein: 9g

Ingredients

2 cups milk (dairy free)

2 bananas (frozen or fresh)

2 tablespoons sunflower seeds

¼ cup pitted dates (about 4 dates)

juice of 4 limes

zest of 4 limes

½ teaspoon pure vanilla extract

2 - 4 drops lime therapeutic grade essential oils, (optional)

1 cup mango

Preparation Method

Blend the sunflower seeds, dates, and some milk first, and form a thick mixture. Add more milk along with the remaining ingredients. Blend for a couple of minutes until the mixture forms a thick, creamy smoothie.

Serve with ice and enjoy fresh!

Fruity Mango Blend

With no more than four ingredients, this fruity smoothie is a terrific blend to fill you up. Enjoy the delicious flavors of this creamy blend that has several health benefits to offer you, including successful weight loss.

Nutritional Values per Serving

Calories: 260

Total Fat: 2g

Carbohydrates: 31g

Protein: 4g

Ingredients

2 cups milk (dairy free)

1 cup spinach

1 cup oats

2 cups mango (chopped, fresh or frozen)

Preparation Method

Blend spinach and milk together in a high-speed blender for a few minutes until it is in liquid form. Add the remaining ingredients and blend again for several minutes until the mixture is thick and creamy.

Add ice cubes in the end, and give it one final blend. Serve fresh and enjoy fresh!

Minty Pineapple Smoothie

The combination of pineapple and mint makes this smoothie one of the most delicious blends!

Nutritional Values per Serving

Calories: 226

Total Fat: 3g

Carbohydrates: 48g

Protein: 5g

Ingredients

1 cup water

4 cups pineapple

2 cups bananas (fresh or frozen)

10 mint leaves

2 tablespoons flaxseeds/linseeds

1 drop mint therapeutic grade essential oil, (optional)

Preparation Method

Blend mint leaves, flaxseeds/linseeds, and water together until it is in liquid form. Add the remaining ingredients, and blend again for several minutes until it forms a thick smoothie.

Adjust the consistency of your smoothie by adding more water if you like. Add ice, and pour in a glass to serve fresh immediately.

Vitamin C Cocktail Smoothie

The blend of the all the ingredients in this recipe has shown great results for weight loss for a very long time. This could help you get weight loss you want by following a vitamin C-loaded smoothie recipe. Prepare yourself!

Nutritional Values per Serving

Calories: 145

Total Fat: 4.7g

Carbohydrates: 29g

Protein: 2g

Ingredients

2 oranges

1 cup strawberries

½ cantaloupe

1 tomato

Preparation Method

Juice the oranges first, and then blend them with the remaining ingredients. Add ice if you want to enjoy this chilled. Serve immediately, and enjoy the refreshing flavors of this delicious smoothie!

Green Tropical Thick Smoothie

This green thick smoothie is easy to prepare. The blend of fruits, vegetables, and seeds will provide your body with all the essential nutrients that you need in order to lose weight and boost your metabolism.

Nutritional Values per Serving

Calories: 251

Total Fat: 10g

Carbohydrates: 33g

Protein: 6g

Ingredients

1 cup water

1½ cups cantaloupe melon

2 cups pineapple

1 cup banana

1 cup spinach

2 tablespoons sunflower seeds

½ cup coconut milk

1 cup oats

Preparation Method

Blend the spinach with water first. Add all the remaining ingredients next, and blend at high for several minutes until it forms a creamy mixture.

Pour into a glass, and add ice cubes. Serve chilled for best flavors.

Chocolate and Marzipan Smoothie

Enjoy the chocolaty-flavored smoothie with the nutrients of fruits, nuts, and vegetables. The unique blend is surely a great addition to your weight loss diet.

Nutritional Values per Serving

Calories: 320

Total Fat: 12g

Carbohydrates: 8g

Protein: 2g

Ingredients

2 cups almond milk (or any other dairy free milk)

1 cup mango (chopped)

¼ cup ground almonds

6 tablespoons cocoa or carob powder

¼ cup pitted dates (about 4 dates)

1 teaspoon almond extract

2 tablespoons almond butter

1 cup oats

1 cup spinach

Preparation Method

Blend spinach and almond milk first. Add all the remaining ingredients in the blender, and pulse at high until everything is smooth.

Pour into a glass, and set into your freezer for 10 minutes before serving.

Super Blue Magic

Loaded with nutrients of blueberries, this three-ingredient smoothie will serve your taste buds like no other.

Nutritional Values per Serving

Calories: 273

Total Fat: 14.5g

Carbohydrates: 29g

Protein:9g

Ingredients

1 cup milk (dairy free)

1 cup blueberries (unsweetened, frozen)

1 tablespoon cold-pressed organic flaxseed oil

Preparation Method

Combine blueberries with milk in a high-speed blender. and pulse for 1 minute. When done, pour into a glass, and stir in flaxseed oil.

Set to chill for some time before drinking for enhanced flavors.

Choco-Raspberry Smoothie

If you are a fan of chocolate and berries, this is the perfect blend for. Try it out yourself!

Nutritional Values per Serving

Calories: 432

Total Fat: 13.5g

Carbohydrates: 77g

Protein: 16g

Ingredients

½ cup soy milk (or any other dairy free milk)

6 oz. vanilla fat-free yogurt

1 cup raspberries (fresh)

¼ cup chocolate chips (unsweetened, dairy free)

A handful frozen raspberries

Preparation Method

Place all the ingredients in a blender, and pulse at high until smooth, for around 1 minute. Transfer the smoothie to a glass, and enjoy the refreshing flavors of this special weight-loss smoothie.

Blueberry and Vanilla Yogurt Smoothie

Delicious blueberries are once again combined with the flavors of vanilla to give you a refreshing smoothie rich in essential nutrients for health and weight loss.

Nutritional Values per Serving

Calories: 443

Total Fat: 14.5g

Carbohydrates: 63g

Protein: 18g

Ingredients

1 cup soy milk (or any other dairy free milk)

6 oz. vanilla fat-free yogurt

1 cup blueberries (fresh)

1 tablespoon flaxseed oil

a handful frozen blueberries

Preparation Method

Place milk, fresh blueberries, yogurt, and frozen blueberries in a blender and pulse at high for a minute until it forms a smooth mixture.

Pour it into a glass, and stir in flaxseed oil before serving it. Drink immediately for best flavors.

Peachy Pour Smoothie

The simple peach-flavored smoothie will take as little as three ingredients to make the nutrient-loaded recipe!

Nutritional Values per Serving

Calories: 213

Total Fat: 9g

Carbohydrates: 26g

Protein: 9g

Ingredients

1 cup milk (dairy free)

1 cup peaches (unsweetened, frozen)

2 tsp cold-pressed organic flaxseed oil

Preparation Method

Combine peaches and milk together in a blender, pulsing it at high for a minute until smooth. Transfer to a glass, and stir in the flaxseed oil. Add ice cubes, and enjoy this fruity smoothie.

Citrusy Smoothie

If you like citrusy flavors, you definitely want to add this recipe to your diet plan. This Citrusy Smoothie holds all the essential nutrients for you along with its superb taste.

Nutritional Values per Serving

Calories: 420

Total Fat: 14g

Carbohydrates: 57g

Protein: 18g

Ingredients

1 cup soy milk (or any other dairy free milk)

6 oz. lemon fat-free yogurt

1 medium-sized orange (cleaned, peeled, sliced into sections)

1 cup ice

1 tablespoon flaxseed oil

Preparation Method

Combine yogurt, milk, ice, and orange in a blender and pulse at high for around 1 minute. When done, transfer to a glass, and stir in flaxseed oil. Enjoy immediately.

Green Apple Refresher

The delicious blend of flavors and nutrients makes this smoothie a true health refresher!

Nutritional Values per Serving

Calories: 482

Total Fat: 16.5g

Carbohydrates: 71g

Protein: 19g

Ingredients

½ cup soy milk (or any other dairy free milk)

6 oz. vanilla fat-free yogurt

1 teaspoon apple pie spice

1 medium-sized apple (chopped, peeled)

2 tablespoons cashew butter

1 cup ice

Preparation Method

Combine all the ingredients in a high speed blender for around 1 minute until creamy. Pour into a glass, and stir before drinking fresh.

Berrylicious Smoothie

Love those brightly colored strawberries? If yes, then this is the perfect smoothie for you. Rich in antioxidants and nutrients that boost metabolism, Berrylicious Smoothie is your ultimate choice for a weight-loss plan!

Nutritional Values per Serving

Calories: 216

Total Fat: 9.5g

Carbohydrates: 26g

Protein: 9g

Ingredients

1 cup milk (dairy free)

1 cup strawberries (unsweetened, frozen)

2 tablespoons cold-press organic flaxseed oil

Preparation Method

Combine milk with strawberries in a high speed blender for around 1 minute. Pour into a glass and stir in oil. Add some crushed ice on the top, and serve immediately.

Mocha Smoothie

Add a shot of espresso, and enjoy the nutrient-dense smoothie.

Nutritional Values per Serving

Calories: 251

Total Fat: 8.4g

Carbohydrates: 36g

Protein: 7g

Ingredients

½ cup vanilla frozen fat-free yogurt

2 teaspoons cocoa powder

1 shot espresso

1 cup ice cubes

Preparation Method

Place all the ingredients in a blender, and pulse at high speed for around a minute until smooth. Pour in a glass and serve chilled.

Bright Watermelon Blend

This refreshing blend of watermelon and lemon sherbet is a weight-loss smoothie formula super hit!

Nutritional Values per Serving

Calories: 215

Total Fat: 8.5g

Carbohydrates: 38g

Protein: 9g

Ingredients

6 cups watermelon (seedless, chopped)

1 cup vanilla fat-free yogurt, or non-fat milk,

1 cup ice cubes

Preparation Method

Place watermelon, low-fat vanilla yogurt or non-fat milk, and ice cubes in a blender and pulse at high for a minute until smooth. Serve immediately, and enjoy the fresh flavors.

Honeydew and Kiwi Green Smoothie

You don't want to miss on the delicious flavors of this green smoothie. Provide yourself with much more than just taste with this amazing blend.

Nutritional Values per Serving

Calories: 198

Total Fat: 7g

Carbohydrates: 20g

Protein: 6g

Ingredients

2 cups honeydew (cubed)

1 Granny Smith apple (chopped)

¼ cup pitted dates (about 4 dates)

1 kiwi fruit (chopped)

1 tablespoon lemon juice

1 cup ice cubes

Preparation Method

Place all the ingredients (except ice) in a high speed blender, and pulse to combine well. Add ice next, and give it one short pulse. Pour in a glass, and enjoy fresh.

A SUGGESTED 7-DAY PLAN SMOOTHIE DIET

Here is a suggested 7-day plan for a smoothie only diet. The ideal consumption is three smoothies per day (breakfast, lunch and dinner). You can drink as much as you like to keep yourself from feeling hungry. Also, feel free to switch them around according to your taste and preferences.

Monday	
Breakfast	Citrusy-Creamy Fat-Burning Smoothie
Lunch	Passion Fruit and Mango Smoothie
Dinner	Rippled Red-Berry Smoothie

Tuesday	
Breakfast	Dreamy-Creamy Green Orange Smoothie
Lunch	Banana Pie and Sweet Potato Smoothie
Dinner	Zucchini Bread Smoothie

Wednesday	
Breakfast	Citrusy-Creamy Fat-Burning Smoothie
Lunch	Pear and Almond Smoothie
Dinner	Frozen Orange and Pineapple Smoothie

Thursday

Breakfast	Spiced Butternut Raw Squash Smoothie
Lunch	Turbo Nutrient-Booster Smoothie
Dinner	Berries and Raw-Buckwheat Smoothie

Friday

Breakfast	Citrusy-Creamy Fat-Burning Smoothie
Lunch	Sweet Romaine Lettuce Smoothie
Dinner	Nutritional Key Lime-Pie Smoothie

Saturday

Breakfast	Fruity Mango Blend
Lunch	Minty Pineapple Smoothie
Dinner	Vitamin C Cocktail Smoothie

Sunday

Breakfast	Citrusy-Creamy Fat-Burning Smoothie
Lunch	Green Tropical Thick Smoothie
Dinner	Chocolate and Marzipan Smoothie

FINAL WORD: THE RIGHT WAY TO A HEALTHIER, LIGHTER YOU!

We hope you've enjoyed all the information we have shared with you in this book.

We highly recommend that you consult a healthcare professional before switching to a smoothie-only diet and replacing all your meals with smoothies. Also, combine your smoothie-only diet with regular exercise for amazing weight loss results.

The recipes shared in this book are tried and tested, and are not only delicious but nutritionally rich to provide your body with all the essential nutrients missed by skipping meals. Try your favorite ones and come up with your own personalized plan that you can follow!

Use the information in this book for your best interest and enjoy the healthy transformation.

Good luck, and great smoothies!